CHRONIC KIDNEY DISEASE

HOW TO ENHANCE KIDNEY FUNCTION AND PREVENT DIALYSIS

DR. AHMED NICOLAS

Table of Contents

CHAPTER ONE

INTRODUCTION TO CHRONIC KIDNEY DISEASE

Chronic Kidney Disease (CKD) poses a significant public health challenge worldwide, affecting millions of individuals and presenting a complex array of medical, social, and economic burdens. Understanding the intricate functions of the kidneys, recognizing the diverse causes and risk factors contributing to CKD, and appreciating the paramount importance of early detection are pivotal in addressing this pervasive health issue.

A. Understanding the Kidneys

The kidneys, though often overlooked in everyday discourse on health, are indispensable organs responsible for a multitude of vital functions within the human body. Situated in the lower back, these bean-shaped organs play a pivotal role in filtering waste products and excess fluids from the blood, regulating electrolyte balance, controlling blood pressure, and producing essential hormones that contribute to red blood cell production and bone health.

The intricate structure of the kidneys comprises millions of tiny filtering units called nephrons, each composed of a glomerulus and a tubule. Blood flows into the glomerulus, where waste products are filtered out and subsequently processed along the tubules, ultimately resulting in the formation of urine. This meticulous filtration process ensures the maintenance of homeostasis within the body, keeping the blood clean and chemically balanced.

B. Causes and Risk Factors of Chronic Kidney Disease

Chronic Kidney Disease can arise from a myriad of factors, both intrinsic and extrinsic, which can compromise the normal functioning of the kidneys over time. Common underlying conditions contributing to CKD include hypertension (high blood pressure) and diabetes mellitus, which exert damaging effects on the delicate blood vessels and nephrons of the kidneys, leading to progressive renal impairment.

Other predisposing factors encompass lifestyle choices such as tobacco use, excessive alcohol consumption, and a diet high in salt and processed foods, all of which can exacerbate kidney dysfunction.

Additionally, certain genetic predispositions and hereditary conditions may render individuals more susceptible to developing CKD, underscoring the intricate interplay between genetic and environmental factors in disease pathogenesis.

C. Importance of Early Detection

Early detection of Chronic Kidney Disease is paramount in mitigating its progression and minimizing associated complications. Unfortunately, CKD often manifests insidiously in its initial stages, with symptoms remaining subtle or absent until significant renal damage has occurred. Routine screening for CKD through simple blood and urine tests can facilitate the timely identification of abnormalities in kidney function, enabling prompt intervention and implementation of therapeutic strategies aimed at preserving renal health.

By emphasizing the significance of early detection and fostering greater awareness of the modifiable risk factors contributing to CKD, efforts can be directed towards preemptive measures aimed at mitigating disease progression and enhancing overall kidney health. Through a comprehensive understanding of the kidneys, recognition of the diverse etiological factors underpinning CKD, and a commitment to proactive screening initiatives, strides can be made towards alleviating the burden of this prevalent and debilitating condition.

CHAPTER TWO

DIAGNOSIS AND STAGES OF
CHRONIC KIDNEY DISEASE

A. Identifying Symptoms

Chronic Kidney Disease often progresses silently, with symptoms manifesting only in advanced stages when significant renal impairment has already occurred. Common symptoms include fatigue, weakness, swelling in the ankles, feet, or hands (edema), difficulty concentrating, decreased appetite, and changes in urination patterns such as increased frequency or decreased volume. However, these symptoms are nonspecific and may overlap with other medical conditions, necessitating a high index of suspicion for CKD, particularly in individuals with known risk factors such as hypertension, diabetes, or a family history of kidney disease.

B. Diagnostic Tests and Procedures

Accurate diagnosis of CKD relies on a combination of clinical evaluation and laboratory investigations. Routine screening tests such as blood pressure measurement, serum creatinine level assessment, and urinalysis are fundamental in identifying individuals at risk or with established CKD. Serum creatinine, a byproduct of muscle metabolism, serves as a surrogate marker of kidney function, with elevated levels indicative of impaired renal clearance.

Additional diagnostic tests may include estimated glomerular filtration rate (eGFR) calculation, which provides an estimate of kidney function based on serum creatinine levels, and imaging studies such as ultrasound or CT scans to evaluate kidney structure and detect any structural abnormalities.

Urinary biomarkers, including albuminuria and proteinuria, are valuable indicators of kidney damage and can aid in risk stratification and prognostication. Microscopic examination of urine sediment may also reveal abnormalities suggestive of underlying renal pathology, further guiding diagnostic and management decisions.

C. Staging and Progression of the Disease

Once diagnosed, CKD is staged based on the severity of renal dysfunction and the presence of kidney damage, as outlined by the Kidney Disease Improving Global Outcomes (KDIGO) guidelines. Staging incorporates both estimated glomerular filtration rate (eGFR) and the degree of albuminuria, categorizing CKD into five stages ranging from mild (Stage 1) to end-stage renal disease (Stage 5).

Each stage is associated with specific management goals and interventions aimed at slowing disease progression and minimizing complications. Regular monitoring of kidney function through serial measurements of eGFR and urinary biomarkers is essential in tracking disease progression and adjusting treatment strategies accordingly.

CHAPTER THREE

LIFESTYLE MODIFICATIONS FOR KIDNEY HEALTH

A. Diet and Nutrition Guidelines

Dietary modifications constitute a cornerstone of kidney health management, with tailored nutrition plans aimed at reducing the burden on the kidneys while providing essential nutrients. Individuals with CKD are often advised to limit their intake of sodium, potassium, and phosphorus, as these electrolytes can accumulate in the body in the setting of impaired renal excretion, leading to electrolyte imbalances and cardiovascular complications.

A balanced diet rich in fruits, vegetables, whole grains, and lean proteins is recommended, emphasizing portion control and moderation of high-protein foods. Dietary restrictions may vary depending on the stage of CKD and individual patient factors, necessitating personalized nutrition counseling from a registered dietitian with expertise in kidney disease management.

B. Importance of Hydration

Proper hydration is essential for maintaining kidney function and promoting optimal urinary output, facilitating the elimination of waste products and toxins from the body. Adequate fluid intake helps prevent the formation of kidney stones and urinary tract infections, common complications in individuals with CKD.

While hydration needs vary depending on individual factors such as age, body weight, and activity level, a general recommendation is to consume sufficient fluids throughout the day, primarily in the form of water. Monitoring urine output and maintaining pale-yellow urine coloration are simple yet effective strategies for assessing hydration status and ensuring adequate fluid intake.

C. Exercise and Physical Activity Recommendations

Regular physical activity confers numerous benefits for kidney health, including improved cardiovascular function, enhanced blood flow to the kidneys, and weight management, all of which contribute to the prevention of CKD progression and associated comorbidities. Exercise also helps alleviate symptoms of fatigue and depression commonly experienced by individuals with CKD, promoting overall quality of life.

Exercise recommendations for individuals with CKD should be tailored to individual capabilities and medical comorbidities, with a focus on low-impact activities such as walking, cycling, swimming, and yoga. Gradual progression and incorporation of both aerobic and resistance training exercises are encouraged, under the guidance of a healthcare professional or certified exercise specialist.

CHAPTER FOUR

MEDICATION MANAGEMENT

A. Overview of Medications for Kidney Disease

The pharmacological management of CKD is multifaceted, addressing various aspects of kidney function and associated comorbidities. Commonly prescribed medications include:

Angiotensin-converting enzyme (ACE) inhibitors and angiotensin II receptor blockers (ARBs): These agents are first-line treatments for managing hypertension in individuals with CKD, exerting renoprotective effects by dilating blood vessels and reducing intraglomerular pressure.

Diuretics: Diuretic therapy may be prescribed to alleviate fluid retention and edema in individuals with CKD, promoting diuresis and reducing extracellular fluid volume.

Erythropoiesis-stimulating agents (ESAs): ESAs are administered to manage anemia associated with CKD by stimulating the production of red blood cells, thereby improving oxygen delivery to tissues and alleviating symptoms of fatigue and weakness.

Phosphate binders: Individuals with CKD often experience hyperphosphatemia due to impaired renal phosphate excretion, necessitating the use of phosphate binders to reduce serum phosphate levels and prevent the development of mineral and bone disorders.

Statins: Statin therapy may be initiated to manage dyslipidemia and reduce cardiovascular risk in individuals with CKD, given the high prevalence of atherosclerotic disease in this population.

B. Managing Blood Pressure and Blood Sugar Levels

Controlling blood pressure and blood sugar levels is paramount in slowing the progression of CKD and reducing the risk of cardiovascular complications. Antihypertensive medications, including ACE inhibitors, ARBs, calcium channel blockers, and beta-blockers, are prescribed to achieve target blood pressure goals and mitigate the detrimental effects of hypertension on kidney function.

For individuals with diabetes, tight glycemic control is essential in preventing diabetic nephropathy and delaying the progression of

CKD. Antidiabetic medications such as insulin, metformin, sulfonylureas, and sodium-glucose cotransporter-2 (SGLT2) inhibitors may be prescribed to optimize blood glucose levels and minimize renal damage.

C. Role of Medications in Slowing Disease Progression

Certain medications have demonstrated efficacy in slowing the progression of CKD and preserving renal function over time. ACE inhibitors and ARBs, in addition to their antihypertensive effects, exert renoprotective effects by reducing intraglomerular pressure and inhibiting the progression of glomerulosclerosis and tubulointerstitial fibrosis.

Furthermore, emerging therapies such as mineralocorticoid receptor antagonists and endothelin receptor antagonists show promise in attenuating renal inflammation and fibrosis, offering potential avenues for targeted intervention in CKD progression.

CHAPTER FIVE

ALTERNATIVE THERAPIES AND COMPLEMENTARY APPROACHES

A. Herbal Remedies and Supplements

Herbal remedies and dietary supplements have long been used in traditional medicine systems worldwide for their purported therapeutic benefits in promoting kidney health and ameliorating symptoms associated with CKD. Commonly utilized herbs and supplements include:

Astragalus: Known for its immune-modulating and anti-inflammatory properties, astragalus is believed to support renal function and improve kidney outcomes in individuals with CKD.

Cordyceps: Derived from a parasitic fungus, cordyceps is purported to enhance renal blood flow, reduce proteinuria, and protect against kidney injury through its antioxidant and anti-inflammatory effects.

Omega-3 fatty acids: Omega-3 supplements, found in fish oil and flaxseed oil, may exert renoprotective effects by reducing inflammation, oxidative stress, and proteinuria in individuals with CKD.

Vitamin D: Vitamin D supplementation is commonly recommended in individuals with CKD to mitigate the risk of bone mineral disorders and reduce secondary hyperparathyroidism.

While herbal remedies and supplements hold promise as adjunctive therapies for CKD management, their efficacy and safety profiles require further investigation through rigorous clinical trials and research studies to elucidate their role in the treatment paradigm.

B. Acupuncture and Traditional Chinese Medicine

Acupuncture, a key component of Traditional Chinese Medicine (TCM), involves the insertion of fine needles into specific points on the body to stimulate therapeutic effects and restore energy balance. In the context of CKD, acupuncture may alleviate symptoms such as pain, fatigue, and nausea, while also improving overall well-being and quality of life.

TCM approaches to CKD management often incorporate herbal medicine, dietary therapy, acupuncture, and lifestyle modifications to address underlying imbalances in the body and promote kidney health. By restoring harmony between the body's organ systems, TCM aims to optimize renal function and slow the progression of CKD.

C. Mindfulness and Stress Reduction Techniques

Mindfulness-based stress reduction techniques, including meditation, deep breathing exercises, and yoga, offer valuable tools for managing stress, anxiety, and depression commonly experienced by individuals with CKD. These practices promote relaxation, improve emotional resilience, and enhance coping mechanisms, thereby contributing to better psychological and physiological outcomes in CKD patients.

By cultivating mindfulness and incorporating stress reduction techniques into daily routines, individuals with CKD can reduce the burden of psychological distress, enhance their sense of well-being, and improve their ability to cope with the challenges of living with a chronic illness.

CHAPTER SIX

DIALYSIS OPTIONS AND CONSIDERATIONS

A. Understanding Dialysis Treatment

Dialysis treatment functions as an artificial replacement for impaired kidney function, replicating the filtration and excretory processes of the kidneys to maintain biochemical equilibrium and fluid balance within the body. By utilizing specialized equipment and dialysis solutions, dialysis therapy removes waste products, toxins, and excess fluid from the bloodstream, thereby alleviating symptoms of uremia and mitigating the complications of kidney failure.

Two primary modalities of dialysis are commonly employed: hemodialysis and peritoneal dialysis. Each modality has distinct advantages, considerations, and implications for patient management, necessitating individualized treatment plans tailored to patient preferences, clinical status, and lifestyle factors.

B. Types of Dialysis: Hemodialysis vs. Peritoneal Dialysis

Hemodialysis: Hemodialysis involves the extracorporeal removal of waste products and excess fluid from the blood using a hemodialysis machine and an artificial semipermeable membrane (dialyzer). During hemodialysis sessions, blood is withdrawn from the patient's vascular access site, circulated through the dialyzer, and returned to the patient's bloodstream after purification. Hemodialysis is typically performed in a dialysis center under the supervision of trained healthcare professionals, with sessions lasting several hours and occurring multiple times per week.

Peritoneal Dialysis: Peritoneal dialysis utilizes the peritoneal membrane lining the abdominal cavity as a natural semipermeable membrane for fluid and solute exchange. During peritoneal dialysis, a dialysis solution (dialysate) is instilled into the peritoneal cavity via a catheter, allowing waste products and excess fluid to diffuse across the peritoneal membrane into the dialysate. Following a dwell time, the used dialysate is drained from the peritoneal cavity, and fresh dialysate is instilled for subsequent cycles. Peritoneal dialysis offers greater flexibility and autonomy, as it can be performed at home by the patient or caregiver, reducing the need for frequent clinic visits

C. Preparation and Maintenance for Dialysis

Preparation for dialysis entails comprehensive education, vascular access placement, and psychosocial support to facilitate the transition to renal replacement therapy. Patients undergoing hemodialysis require vascular access for blood withdrawal and return, typically achieved through arteriovenous fistulas, arteriovenous grafts, or central venous catheters. Adequate vascular access is crucial for ensuring optimal dialysis efficiency and minimizing complications such as infection and thrombosis.

In contrast, patients opting for peritoneal dialysis undergo surgical implantation of a peritoneal dialysis catheter, which serves as the conduit for dialysis solution instillation and drainage. Careful attention to catheter care, infection prevention, and peritoneal hygiene is essential to optimize peritoneal dialysis outcomes and minimize the risk of peritonitis and catheter-related complications.

Regular monitoring, adherence to dietary and fluid restrictions, and compliance with prescribed medications are integral aspects of dialysis maintenance, ensuring optimal treatment efficacy and patient well-being. Additionally, ongoing support from multidisciplinary healthcare teams, including nephrologists, dialysis nurses, dietitians, and social workers, is essential in addressing the multifaceted needs of individuals undergoing dialysis therapy.

CHAPTER SEVEN

STRATEGIES FOR ENHANCING KIDNEY FUNCTION

A. Renal Rehabilitation Programs

Renal rehabilitation programs provide comprehensive, multidisciplinary interventions tailored to the unique needs of individuals with CKD, offering a holistic approach to kidney health management. These programs typically involve coordinated efforts from healthcare professionals, including nephrologists, nurses, dietitians, physical therapists, and social workers, to address the multifaceted aspects of CKD care.

Components of renal rehabilitation programs may include:

Dietary and Nutritional Counseling: Guidance on adopting a kidney-friendly diet low in sodium, potassium, and phosphorus, while emphasizing the importance of adequate protein intake and hydration.

Exercise and Physical Activity: Structured exercise programs aimed at improving cardiovascular fitness, muscle strength, and overall physical function, tailored to individual capabilities and preferences.

Medication Management: Optimization of medication regimens to control blood pressure, manage blood sugar levels, and alleviate symptoms associated with CKD, while minimizing adverse effects and drug interactions.

Psychosocial Support: Counseling and support services to address emotional and psychological challenges associated with living with CKD, including stress, anxiety, depression, and adjustment to lifestyle changes.

Renal rehabilitation programs empower individuals with CKD to actively participate in their care, fostering self-management skills and promoting adherence to recommended treatment regimens. By addressing modifiable risk factors, optimizing medical management, and promoting lifestyle modifications, these programs play a pivotal role in enhancing kidney function and improving outcomes for individuals with CKD.

B. Therapeutic Approaches to Kidney Repair

Therapeutic approaches to kidney repair focus on harnessing the regenerative potential of renal tissue to stimulate repair mechanisms and restore normal kidney function. These approaches encompass a variety of strategies, including:

Cell-Based Therapies: Stem cell therapy and regenerative medicine techniques hold promise for promoting renal regeneration and repairing damaged nephrons. Stem cells derived from various sources, including bone marrow, adipose tissue, and umbilical cord blood, have been investigated for their potential to differentiate into renal progenitor cells and promote tissue repair.

Gene Therapy: Gene editing technologies such as CRISPR-Cas9 offer novel opportunities for correcting genetic mutations underlying inherited kidney disorders and promoting renal regeneration. By targeting specific genes implicated in renal disease pathogenesis, gene therapy holds potential for mitigating disease progression and restoring normal kidney function.

Tissue Engineering: Tissue engineering approaches involve the fabrication of bioengineered renal constructs using biomaterials and cell-based therapies, with the goal of developing functional kidney tissue for transplantation or implantation. These bioengineered constructs mimic the structure and function of native kidney tissue, offering potential solutions for renal replacement therapy and organ regeneration.

C. Emerging Technologies and Research in Kidney Regeneration

Emerging technologies and research in kidney regeneration are driving advances in the field of nephrology, offering innovative approaches for enhancing kidney function and promoting renal repair. Key areas of focus include:

Organoids and Organ-on-a-Chip Models: 3D organoid cultures and microfluidic organ-on-a-chip models provide valuable tools for studying kidney development, disease mechanisms, and drug screening in a controlled laboratory setting. These models recapitulate the complexity of native kidney tissue, enabling researchers to investigate disease pathogenesis and explore potential therapeutic interventions.

Bioprinting: 3D bioprinting technologies enable the fabrication of intricate renal structures using bioink formulations containing living cells and biomaterials. Bioprinted kidney constructs can be customized to mimic the architecture and function of native kidney tissue, offering potential solutions for organ transplantation and tissue regeneration.

Nanomedicine: Nanotechnology-based approaches hold promise for targeted drug delivery, imaging, and diagnostic applications in kidney disease management. Nanoparticle-based drug delivery systems can enhance drug bioavailability, reduce systemic toxicity, and improve therapeutic efficacy in CKD treatment.

CHAPTER EIGHT

PREVENTIVE MEASURES AND FUTURE OUTLOOK

A. Preventing Complications and Disease Progression

Preventive measures play a central role in mitigating the risk of complications and slowing the progression of CKD, thereby preserving renal function and reducing the burden of kidney disease. Key strategies include:

Blood Pressure Control: Tight blood pressure control is essential in slowing the progression of CKD and reducing the risk of cardiovascular complications. Lifestyle modifications, including dietary sodium restriction, regular exercise, and medication adherence, are cornerstone interventions in managing hypertension in individuals with CKD.

Blood Sugar Management: Individuals with diabetes are at increased risk of developing CKD and progressing to ESRD. Optimal glycemic control through dietary modifications, physical activity, and antidiabetic medications is crucial in preventing diabetic nephropathy and delaying CKD progression.

Smoking Cessation: Tobacco use is a modifiable risk factor for CKD progression and cardiovascular disease. Smoking cessation interventions, including behavioral counseling, pharmacotherapy, and support services, are essential in reducing the risk of kidney damage and improving overall health outcomes.

Dietary Modifications: Adopting a kidney-friendly diet low in sodium, potassium, and phosphorus, while emphasizing adequate protein intake and hydration, can help mitigate the risk of complications such as electrolyte imbalances, fluid overload, and mineral and bone disorders in individuals with CKD.

B. Importance of Regular Monitoring and Follow-up

Regular monitoring and follow-up are essential components of CKD management, enabling early detection of complications, timely intervention, and optimization of treatment strategies. Key elements of regular monitoring include:

Kidney Function Tests: Serial measurements of serum creatinine, estimated glomerular filtration rate (eGFR), and urinary biomarkers such as albuminuria and proteinuria provide valuable insights into renal function and disease progression.

Blood Pressure Monitoring: Regular blood pressure measurements are essential in assessing hypertension control and guiding antihypertensive therapy adjustments to achieve target blood pressure goals.

Medication Review: Periodic medication reviews ensure optimal pharmacotherapy management, minimize polypharmacy, and reduce the risk of drug-induced nephrotoxicity and adverse effects.

Regular communication and collaboration between patients, healthcare providers, and multidisciplinary care teams are essential in facilitating comprehensive CKD management and promoting patient engagement and adherence to recommended treatment regimens.

C. Promising Advances in Kidney Disease Treatment

Promising advances in kidney disease treatment offer hope for improved outcomes and enhanced quality of life for individuals with CKD. Key areas of innovation and research include:

Precision Medicine: Advances in genomic medicine and personalized medicine approaches hold promise for identifying genetic risk factors, predicting disease progression, and tailoring treatment strategies to individual patient characteristics.

Renal Replacement Therapies: Innovations in dialysis technology, including wearable and portable dialysis devices, offer opportunities for enhanced convenience, flexibility, and autonomy for individuals requiring renal replacement therapy.

Regenerative Medicine: Stem cell therapy, tissue engineering, and regenerative medicine approaches hold potential for promoting renal regeneration, repairing damaged nephrons, and restoring normal kidney function in individuals with CKD.

Biomedical Engineering: Biomaterials, nanotechnology, and bioengineering innovations offer novel solutions for targeted drug delivery, imaging, and diagnostic applications in kidney disease management, facilitating early detection, and intervention.

CHAPTER NINE

LIVING WELL WITH CHRONIC KIDNEY DISEASE

A. Coping Strategies and Emotional Support

Coping with the physical and emotional toll of CKD requires the implementation of effective coping strategies and access to emotional support systems. Key coping strategies include:

Education and Empowerment: Understanding the nature of CKD, its treatment options, and lifestyle modifications empowers individuals to actively participate in their care and make informed decisions.

Social Support: Building a strong support network of family, friends, peers, and support groups provides emotional validation, encouragement, and practical assistance in coping with the challenges of CKD.

Mindfulness and Stress Reduction: Engaging in mindfulness-based practices, relaxation techniques, and stress reduction activities such as meditation, deep breathing exercises, and yoga can alleviate anxiety, promote emotional well-being, and enhance coping mechanisms.

Seeking Professional Help: Consulting with mental health professionals, counselors, or therapists can provide additional support in managing emotional distress, depression, and adjustment issues related to living with CKD.

B. Maintaining Quality of Life

Maintaining quality of life while living with CKD involves addressing physical, emotional, social, and spiritual dimensions of well-being. Strategies for enhancing quality of life include:

Adherence to Treatment Regimens: Strict adherence to prescribed medication regimens, dietary modifications, and lifestyle recommendations is essential in managing CKD, preventing complications, and optimizing overall health outcomes.

Physical Activity and Exercise: Incorporating regular physical activity and exercise into daily routines promotes cardiovascular health, muscle strength, and mobility, while also alleviating symptoms of fatigue and depression commonly associated with CKD.

Nutritional Support: Following a kidney-friendly diet low in sodium, potassium, and phosphorus, while emphasizing adequate protein intake and hydration, supports renal function, mitigates complications, and enhances overall well-being.

Engagement in Meaningful Activities: Pursuing hobbies, interests, and activities that bring joy, fulfillment, and a sense of purpose fosters a positive outlook, reduces stress, and enhances overall quality of life.

C. Resources and Supportive Services for Patients and Caregivers

Access to resources and supportive services is essential in providing comprehensive care and addressing the diverse needs of individuals with CKD and their caregivers. Key resources and supportive services include:

Patient Education Programs: Educational materials, workshops, and classes offered through healthcare providers, hospitals, and community organizations provide valuable information on CKD management, treatment options, and self-care strategies.

Support Groups: Peer-led support groups, online forums, and virtual communities offer opportunities for individuals with CKD and their caregivers to connect, share experiences, and receive emotional support from others facing similar challenges.

Social Services: Social workers, case managers, and patient navigators can provide assistance with navigating healthcare systems, accessing financial resources, coordinating care, and addressing psychosocial needs.

Caregiver Support: Caregiver support services, respite care programs, and caregiver education and training initiatives help alleviate caregiver burden, provide practical assistance, and promote caregiver well-being in caring for individuals with CKD.

CHAPTER TEN

CONCLUSION:

EMPOWERING YOURSELF FOR
KIDNEY HEALTH

Empowering yourself for kidney health is a transformative journey that involves taking charge of your health, embracing hope for the future, and thriving despite the challenges posed by Chronic Kidney Disease (CKD). By adopting a proactive approach to kidney health management, leveraging support systems, and cultivating resilience, individuals with CKD can enhance their well-being, optimize treatment outcomes, and lead fulfilling lives.

A. Taking Charge of Your Health Journey

Taking charge of your health journey begins with self-awareness, education, and empowerment. By understanding the nature of CKD, its risk factors, and management strategies, individuals can make informed decisions, advocate for their needs, and actively participate in their care. Key steps in taking charge of your health journey include:

Self-Advocacy: Speaking up, asking questions, and expressing concerns during healthcare interactions empowers individuals to assert their preferences, voice their goals, and collaborate with healthcare providers in developing personalized treatment plans.

Self-Management: Implementing self-care strategies, adhering to treatment regimens, and monitoring health indicators empower individuals to take control of their health, mitigate complications, and optimize overall well-being.

Lifestyle Modifications: Making healthy lifestyle choices, including maintaining a balanced diet, engaging in regular physical activity, managing stress, and avoiding harmful habits such as smoking, supports kidney health and improves quality of life.

By embracing a proactive and empowered approach to kidney health, individuals with CKD can navigate the complexities of their condition with confidence, resilience, and a sense of empowerment.

B. Hope for the Future: Thriving Despite Chronic Kidney Disease

Despite the challenges posed by CKD, there is hope for the future. With advancements in medical research, innovative treatments, and supportive care initiatives, individuals with CKD can envision a future filled with possibilities, resilience, and hope. Key aspects of fostering hope for the future include:

Advancements in Treatment: Promising developments in kidney disease treatment, including regenerative medicine, precision medicine, and novel therapeutic approaches, offer hope for improved outcomes, enhanced quality of life, and potential cures for CKD in the future.

Supportive Care Initiatives: Access to resources, support services, and multidisciplinary care teams provides individuals with CKD and their caregivers with the tools, guidance, and assistance needed to navigate the challenges of their condition, manage symptoms, and optimize well-being.

Community Engagement: Engaging with peer support groups, advocacy organizations, and community networks fosters a sense of belonging, solidarity, and shared experiences, empowering individuals with CKD to connect, share stories, and draw strength from one another.

By embracing hope for the future, individuals with CKD can transcend the limitations of their condition, cultivate resilience, and thrive despite the obstacles they may encounter along their journey to kidney health.

In conclusion, empowering yourself for kidney health involves taking charge of your health journey, embracing hope for the future, and recognizing the resilience and strength within yourself. By advocating for your needs, making informed decisions, and fostering a sense of hope and optimism, you can navigate the complexities of Chronic Kidney Disease with grace, resilience, and a sense of empowerment. Individuals with CKD can take proactive steps towards enhancing kidney function, preserving renal health, and ultimately, preventing the need for dialysis. With dedication, perseverance, and the support of healthcare providers, family, and community networks, individuals with CKD can embark on a journey towards improved renal outcomes and a higher quality of life.